SJOGREN'S SYNDROME DIET COOKBOOK:

FOR NEWLY DIAGNOSED

Complete Beginner Procedures, Food Recipes, Guided Meal Plans, And Healthy Lifestyle Tips To Manage, Strive And Live Well With Sjogren's Syndrome

DR. EMMY BROOKS

ABOUT THIS BOOK

The "Sjogren's Syndrome Diet Cookbook" stands as an invaluable guide, seamlessly blending comprehensive knowledge with practical applications to empower individuals grappling with Sjogren's Syndrome. In the introduction, the book establishes a solid foundation, delving into the intricate relationship between Sjogren's Syndrome and nutrition, illuminating the essential role a customized diet plays in managing this challenging condition.

Chapter by chapter, the book unfolds like a culinary odyssey, each section meticulously crafted to equip readers with the knowledge and tools needed to navigate the complexities of Sjogren's-friendly eating. Chapter One carefully unveils the nature of Sjogren's Syndrome, shedding light on its symptoms and the profound impact it can have on daily life. The subsequent chapters seamlessly build upon this understanding, exploring the foundations of a diet tailored to Sjogren's and offering practical advice on ingredient choices and cooking techniques.

The heart of the book lies in its diverse and delectable recipes, carefully curated to not only delight the palate but also serve as powerful allies in managing symptoms. From breakfast options like the Berry Bliss Smoothie and Ginger Turmeric Oatmeal to nutrient-rich lunch ideas and satisfying dinners designed for symptom relief, each recipe is a testament to the belief that flavorful meals can be both healing and enjoyable.

Beyond the kitchen, the book extends its reach into holistic lifestyle habits in Chapter Thirteen, encouraging readers to incorporate mindful practices into their daily lives. The inclusion of a practical meal plan in Chapter Eleven and prep tips for novices in Chapter Twelve further elevates the book's practicality, making it an indispensable companion for those navigating the challenges of Sjogren's Syndrome.

Therefore, "Sjogren's Syndrome Diet Cookbook" is more than a collection of recipes; it's a roadmap for reclaiming control over one's health journey. Empowering and elevating, this book stands as a beacon of support for Sjogren's warriors, guiding them towards a life of nourishment, balance, and joy.

DISCLAIMER:

This book's content is solely intended for general informative purposes. About the availability, applicability, correctness, completeness, and trustworthiness of the data or recipes in this book, the author provides no guarantees of any sort, either stated or implied. You bear full responsibility for any reliance you may have on such material.

The advice, diagnosis, or treatment provided by a qualified medical expert is not to be replaced by this cookbook. When in doubt about a medical problem, never hesitate to consult your doctor or another trained healthcare professional. Never ignore medical advice from professionals or put off getting it because of something you've read in this book.

At the time of publishing, the author of this book has taken reasonable steps to guarantee that the information is correct and current. He does not, however, guarantee that the data will be error-free or that it will satisfy any certain performance or quality standards. Any negative repercussions that may arise from using or applying the material in this book are not the responsibility of the author, publisher, or distributor.

In this book, references or mentions of individuals, products, websites, organizations, or other names are for informational purposes only and do not imply endorsement or affiliation with the author. The author has no control over the nature, content, and availability of referenced or mentioned entities. Any reliance on such information is at the reader's own risk.

The inclusion of any references does not necessarily imply a recommendation or endorse the views expressed within them. The author or publisher shall not be liable for any loss or damage arising out of or in connection with, the use of this book.

INTRODUCTION

Understanding Sjogren's Syndrome And Nutrition

Understanding Sjogren's syndrome and nutrition is crucial for individuals grappling with this autoimmune disorder. Sjogren's syndrome primarily targets the exocrine glands, leading to diminished moisture production in areas such as the eyes and mouth. This persistent dryness can significantly impact daily life, from basic activities like speaking and chewing to broader issues such as compromised nutritional intake and overall well-being.

In the context of Sjogren's Syndrome, nutrition plays a pivotal role in symptom management and enhancing the effectiveness of medical treatments. The focus of a Sjogren's-friendly diet revolves around addressing dryness, supporting the immune system, and combating inflammation – key elements in managing the condition.

Hydration is paramount in mitigating dryness associated with Sjogren's. Adequate water intake, complemented by hydrating foods like watermelon and cucumber, helps alleviate discomfort. Additionally, incorporating omega-3 fatty acids from sources like fatty fish and flaxseeds aids in reducing inflammation, a common feature of autoimmune conditions.

Antioxidant-rich foods, including berries and leafy greens, contribute to immune system support and counteract oxidative stress. These dietary adjustments may initially seem overwhelming, but a step-by-step approach can simplify the process for novices. Gradually introducing changes, such as increasing water intake and experimenting with omega-3-rich foods, allows individuals to adapt without feeling inundated.

Personalization is key in Sjogren's Syndrome and Nutrition equation. Through trial and error, individuals can identify which foods positively Impact their symptoms, tailoring their diet to their unique needs. This not only enhances the efficacy of symptom management but also makes the dietary adjustments sustainable and enjoyable.

In essence, understanding Sjogren's Syndrome and nutrition involves recognizing the link between dietary choices and symptom alleviation. By embracing a tailored approach to nutrition, individuals can empower themselves in the ongoing management of Sjogren's, fostering a sense of control over their well-being and quality of life.

CHAPTER ONE

UNVEILING SJOGREN'S SYNDROME

Overview of Symptoms and Impact on Daily Life

Sjogren's Syndrome is an autoimmune disease that mostly affects the exocrine glands, which reduces the body's ability to produce moisture in many areas, most notably the mouth and eyes. The main signs and symptoms are dry mouth, dry eyes, and trouble swallowing. In addition to these, patients could feel drained and have joint discomfort and increased light sensitivity. Sjogren's affects mental and emotional health in addition to causing physical discomfort, which influences day-to-day living. It may become difficult to chew, speak, or even taste as a result of the ongoing dryness. This not only affects dietary intake but also makes it difficult to do everyday tasks like having a meal or having a conversation.

Apart from the physical symptoms, people with Sjogren's Syndrome frequently struggle with the emotional impact of having a long-term illness. Having to constantly manage symptoms, making numerous doctor's appointments, and not knowing when a flare-up may occur all lead to more stress and anxiety. This intricate interplay of symptoms emphasizes the necessity of treating the illness holistically, emphasizing both medication therapies and lifestyle modifications.

A Customized Diet Is Essential for Managing the Illness

It is impossible to exaggerate how important nutrition is to managing Sjogren's syndrome. A well-designed food plan can improve general health, reduce symptoms, and increase the efficacy of medical interventions. A customized diet for Sjogren largely targets the problems caused by dryness, strengthens the immune system, and reduces inflammation. People can see a major increase in their quality of life by consuming particular nutrients and foods that support these goals.

Staying hydrated is essential for the Sjogren's Syndrome diet. Adequate water intake is crucial because dryness is the main cause of concern. But being hydrated doesn't only mean drinking water—eating foods high in water content, such as fruits and vegetables, is also crucial. These include things like watermelon, cucumbers, and celery, which are high in vitamins and minerals and also help you stay hydrated overall.

Omega-3 fatty acids, which are recognized for their anti-inflammatory qualities, are another essential element. Omega-3-rich foods, such as walnuts, flaxseeds, and fatty fish (salmon, mackerel, and sardines), can help reduce inflammation linked to autoimmune diseases like Sjogren's syndrome. Antioxidant-rich foods, such as kale, spinach, and berries, help to manage symptoms overall by boosting the immune system and preventing oxidative stress.

While implementing these nutritional changes might initially appear intimidating, it can be made more approachable for beginners by breaking it down into smaller steps. One or two little adjustments at a time, such as drinking more water or including foods high in omega-3s in meals, help people adjust to the new eating patterns without feeling overwhelmed.

Making these dietary adjustments enjoyable and durable is crucial. Try several recipes that fit Sjogren's diet to give some variety and make the shift more bearable. With time, people can learn which foods have a beneficial effect on their symptoms and adjust their diets appropriately, developing a customized strategy for using nutrition to manage Sjogren's Syndrome.

CHAPTER TWO

FOUNDATIONS OF A DIET FRIENDLY TO SJOGREN'S

Crucial Elements for the Control of Symptoms:

To properly control their symptoms, people with Sjögren's syndrome must eat a diet rich in nutrients and well-balanced. The first step in creating a diet that is Sjögren's disease-friendly is figuring out which vital elements are most important for managing symptoms.

Because of their anti-inflammatory qualities, omega-3 fatty acids are one of the essential ingredients. Fatty fish like trout, mackerel, and salmon contain these fatty acids. By consuming these fish, you can improve the general health of your joints and tissues and reduce the inflammation brought on by Sjögren's syndrome.

Another important component that people with Sjögren's syndrome should focus on is antioxidants. Selenium, zinc, and vitamins A, C, and E work as potent antioxidants to protect the body from oxidative stress. A robust supply of these antioxidants can be obtained by including colorful fruits and vegetables including bell peppers, spinach, citrus fruits, and berries.

For Sjögren's patients, who frequently feel dry lips and eyes, staying hydrated is essential. Maintaining the body's moisture levels during the day is facilitated by drinking plenty of water. Herbal teas and sugar-free drinks can also be added to offer some variation and boost overall hydration.

For healthy bones, calcium and vitamin D are essential, particularly for those with Sjögren's syndrome who may be more susceptible to osteoporosis. Good sources of calcium include dairy products, fortified plant-based milk, and leafy green vegetables. Moderate sun exposure is necessary for the body to naturally create vitamin D.

Lean protein sources like beans, chicken, and tofu are crucial for maintaining healthy muscles and high energy levels. Sufficient consumption of protein aids in the body's maintenance and repair functions, which is especially advantageous for those with Sjögren's syndrome.

To summarize, a diet that is suitable for people with Sjögren's syndrome should emphasize lean proteins, antioxidants, water, calcium, and vitamin D. Including a range of meals high in nutrients can offer a comprehensive strategy for managing symptoms and promoting general health.

Foods to Take and Leave Out:

To properly manage symptoms, navigating the intricacies of a Sjögren's-friendly diet requires not only recognizing key nutrients but also knowing which foods to include and avoid.

One of the main components of a diet that is Sjögren's-friendly is including a wide range of fruits and vegetables. Cucumbers, celery, berries, and watermelon are hydrating foods that can help maintain the proper balance of moisture in the body.

Furthermore, the oxidative stress linked to the illness can be fought by foods rich in antioxidants, such as kiwis and oranges.

For their omega-3 fatty acids, fatty fish like salmon and sardines should be eaten. These good fats have anti-inflammatory qualities that can help reduce inflammation and joint pain. For best results, try to include these fish in your meals at least twice a week.

Tofu, lentils, and chickpeas are examples of plant-based proteins that provide a protein source without the possible inflammatory effects of some animal proteins. These substitutes can be used in a variety of recipes, giving people who want more diversity in their meals more possibilities.

For the maintenance of bone health, dairy products or dairy substitutes supplemented with calcium and vitamin D are crucial. You should consistently include yogurt, milk, and fortified plant-based milk to ensure that you are getting the required daily intake of these essential nutrients.

Conversely, some foods ought to be avoided or consumed in moderation. Processed foods that are heavy in salt and sugar can aggravate signs of inflammation. Moderation is essential because alcohol and caffeine can also cause dehydration.

It's critical to keep an eye on how your body reacts to different meals and change your diet accordingly. Maintaining a food diary might assist in determining any patterns or triggers that might be impacting your symptoms. Individuals with Sjögren's syndrome can take proactive measures to manage their disease and enhance their overall quality of life by being aware of their food and making educated decisions.

CHAPTER THREE

CONSTRUCTING A HARMONIOUS PLATE

Distribution of Nutrients and Control of Portion:

For people with Sjögren's syndrome, portion control and ensuring adequate distribution of vital nutrients are crucial components of a well-balanced plate. This method promotes general well-being and aids with symptom management.

To start, picture your plate as a canvas with separate parts for each food type. Strive for equilibrium when it comes to healthy fats, proteins, carbs, and a range of vibrant fruits and vegetables. Anti-inflammatory foods can be helpful for people with Sjögren's syndrome.

Start with a source of lean protein, like tofu, fish, or grilled chicken. For the health of your muscles and general energy, you need proteins. For most people, a portion the size of your palm serves as a good guideline, but it's important to take individual needs into account and seek individualized advice from a healthcare provider or dietitian.

Next, set aside some for complex carbohydrates like legumes or whole grains. These are high in fiber, which helps with digestion, and they offer sustained energy. To fill this section of your plate, go for sweet potatoes, brown rice, or quinoa.

Incorporate wholesome fats from foods like nuts, avocados, and olive oil to promote joint health and satiety. Given that fats are high in calories, keep these portions in check. A tiny handful of nuts or a tablespoon of olive oil make a suitable base.

Lastly, arrange a vibrant assortment of vegetables on the remaining area of your plate. Aim for a varied selection because different colors frequently indicate different nutrients. Tomatoes, bell peppers, and leafy greens are great options. These veggies encourage hydration and provide important vitamins and minerals.

Recall that variety and moderation are crucial. Adapt serving sizes to suit individual requirements, activity levels, and any special dietary advice from medical professionals.

Making Filling and Nutritious Meals:

For people with Sjögren's syndrome, creating meals that are both nourishing and satisfying requires carefully balancing flavors, textures, and nutrient-dense ingredients. To prepare meals that please your palate and promote your health, think about these doable steps:

1. Tasty Seasoning: Try different herbs and spices to enhance flavor without using too much salt. Herbs with anti-inflammatory properties, such as basil, cilantro, and mint, also improve flavor.

2. Include Omega-3 Fatty Acids: To increase your intake of omega-3 fatty acids, include fatty fish like salmon or chia seeds in your meals. These are well-known for having anti-inflammatory qualities, making them advantageous for people with autoimmune diseases such as Sjögren's syndrome.

3. Stay Hydrated: Pay attention to foods that are high in water content, as Sjögren's syndrome frequently causes dehydration. Nutritious and hydrating foods include soups, stews, and watery fruits like cucumber and watermelon.

4. Cooking Techniques to Consider: Choose cooking techniques that preserve nutrients without adding too much fat. Grilling, roasting, and steaming are all fantastic options. These techniques support a balanced, healthful diet while preserving the inherent flavors of the ingredients.

5. Fiber-Rich Options: Eat more fruits, vegetables, and whole grains to increase your intake of fiber. Both digestion and blood sugar stability are aided by fiber. Think about including quinoa, brown rice, and an assortment of fresh vegetables in your meals.

6. Protein Variety: To guarantee a well-rounded nutritional profile, change up your sources of protein. Serve lean meats with plant-based proteins like tofu, lentils, and beans. This method adds variety to your diet while also supplying necessary amino acids.

7. Colorful Plate: Try to create a plate that has a range of colors that is visually appealing. This guarantees a variety of nutrients in your meals and also makes them look more appetizing. Diverse hues of fruits and vegetables offer varying compositions of vitamins and minerals.

8. Eat Wisely: Select satiating and nutrient-dense snacks. Slicing veggies with hummus, a handful of nuts, or Greek yogurt with berries are all great combinations. Without sacrificing health, these snacks can support the maintenance of energy levels in between meals.

These simple steps can help you plan meals that are both satisfying and diverse, meeting the unique dietary requirements of people with Sjögren's syndrome. Remember, it's essential to listen to your body and make adjustments based on individual preferences and requirements.

CHAPTER FOUR

ESSENTIAL INGREDIENTS FOR SJOGREN'S-FRIENDLY COOKING

Stocking Your Pantry With Supportive Elements:

Creating a Sjogren 's-friendly pantry is an essential step in ensuring that your cooking aligns with the dietary needs of individuals with Sjogren's Syndrome. Begin by incorporating anti-inflammatory and nutrient-rich staples into your pantry. These include whole grains like quinoa and brown rice, which provide a healthy source of carbohydrates and fiber. Additionally, opt for gluten-free alternatives like almond flour or coconut flour to accommodate those with gluten sensitivities often associated with autoimmune conditions.

Include a variety of nuts and seeds such as walnuts, chia seeds, and flaxseeds, which are rich in omega-3 fatty acids and can contribute to reducing inflammation. Olive oil, with its anti-inflammatory properties, is an excellent choice for cooking and dressing salads. Herbs and spices like turmeric, ginger, and cinnamon can add flavor to your dishes while providing potential anti-inflammatory benefits.

In terms of protein sources, stock up on lean proteins like skinless poultry, fish, and plant-based options such as lentils and beans. Canned beans and legumes are convenient and can be included in various recipes for added protein and fiber. For those looking for dairy alternatives, consider stocking up on almond milk, coconut milk, or other non-dairy options that are fortified with essential nutrients like calcium and vitamin D.

Include a variety of colorful fruits and vegetables, both fresh and frozen, to ensure a diverse range of vitamins and minerals. Berries, leafy greens, and cruciferous vegetables like broccoli and cauliflower are particularly beneficial. Lastly, keep your pantry well-stocked with low-sodium broth, vinegar, and low-sugar canned goods to enhance the flavor of your dishes without compromising on nutritional value.

Smart substitutions for common ingredients:

Making smart substitutions in your cooking is a crucial aspect of adapting to a Sjogren 's-friendly diet. Begin with replacing refined sugars with natural sweeteners like honey, maple syrup, or agave nectar. These alternatives can add sweetness to your dishes without causing spikes in blood sugar levels, which is especially important for those with autoimmune conditions.

Swap out processed and refined grains with whole grains for increased fiber and nutrient content. Brown rice, quinoa, and oats are excellent alternatives that can be seamlessly integrated into various recipes. Consider using gluten-free flours like almond flour, coconut flour, or a blend of gluten-free flours for baking, ensuring that those with gluten sensitivities can still enjoy your culinary creations.

Instead of conventional cooking oils, opt for healthier options like olive oil or avocado oil. These oils not only add flavor but also provide essential fatty acids with potential anti-inflammatory benefits. When choosing dairy products, explore non-dairy alternatives such as almond milk, coconut milk, or oat milk to cater to lactose intolerance or sensitivities.

For seasoning, embrace the vibrant world of herbs and spices. Turmeric, known for its anti-inflammatory properties, can be a great substitute for salt, which should be used sparingly in a Sjogren 's-friendly diet. Experiment with fresh herbs like basil, cilantro, and parsley to enhance the taste of your dishes without relying on excessive salt or unhealthy seasonings.

In recipes calling for red meat, consider leaner protein sources like poultry, fish, or plant-based options. Lentils, chickpeas, and tofu can be used creatively to provide a protein boost without compromising on taste or texture. When it comes to snacks, choose nutrient-dense options like raw nuts, seeds, or fresh fruit instead of processed snacks high in salt and sugar.

By making these smart substitutions, you can create flavorful and satisfying meals that align with the dietary needs of those with Sjogren's Syndrome while promoting overall well-being.

CHAPTER FIVE

SIMPLE AND EFFECTIVE COOKING TECHNIQUES

Cooking Methods for Preserving Nutrients:

Maintaining a nutrient-rich diet is essential for individuals with Sjogren's Syndrome, as it can help alleviate symptoms and promote overall well-being. The cooking methods employed play a crucial role in preserving the nutritional value of ingredients. One of the simplest and most effective techniques is steaming. Steaming vegetables not only retain their vibrant colors but also ensure that water-soluble vitamins like vitamin C remain intact. For a novice, investing in a reliable steamer can make this process hassle-free. Simply chop the vegetables, place them in the steamer basket, and let the gentle steam work its magic.

Another valuable method is stir-frying. This quick and dynamic cooking technique allows you to cook vegetables briefly, preserving their texture and nutritional content. Use a non-stick pan to minimize the need for excessive oils, and opt for heart-healthy options like olive oil.

Stir-frying is not only efficient but also enhances the flavors of your ingredients. Novices can start with a simple stir-fry recipe, incorporating a variety of colorful vegetables for a nutrient-packed dish.

Additionally, roasting is a versatile method that can impart a delightful flavor to proteins and vegetables while preserving their nutritional value. To simplify the process, line a baking sheet with parchment paper, toss your chosen ingredients with a small amount of oil and seasonings, and let the oven do the work. Roasting can bring out the natural sweetness of vegetables and add depth to meats without compromising their nutrient content.

Incorporating these cooking methods into a Sjogren's Syndrome diet ensures that vital nutrients are retained, contributing to a well-balanced and nourishing culinary experience.

Time-Saving Tips for Busy Schedules:

Navigating a busy schedule while adhering to a Sjogren's Syndrome diet requires strategic planning and efficient cooking practices. Batch cooking is a game-changer for those with hectic lifestyles. Dedicate a specific day to preparing large quantities of staple items like grains, proteins, and sauces. Portion them into individual servings and freeze them for later use. This approach not only saves time but also ensures you have nutritious options readily available.

Investing in time-saving kitchen gadgets is another effective strategy. A slow cooker or Instant Pot can be a novice-friendly solution. With minimal effort, you can toss ingredients into the pot in the morning and return to a fully cooked, flavorful meal in the evening. The slow cooking process enhances the depth of flavors while maintaining the nutritional integrity of the ingredients.

Embracing one-pan dishes is a sensible method to streamline your cooking routine. Choose a variety of vegetables, lean proteins, and good grains, toss them together on a baking sheet or in a pan, and let the oven or stovetop do the work. This not only minimizes cleanup but also provides a balanced and time-efficient supper.

For those days when cooking feels daunting, having a repertory of basic dishes is vital. Compile a collection of go-to dishes that require minimal supplies and steps. This may include salads with pre-washed greens, quick stir-fries, or smoothies with frozen fruits and vegetables. The goal is to have solutions that can be prepared in a short amount of time without compromising nutritional content.

By adding these time-saving tips to the Sjogren's Syndrome diet, newbies can handle busy schedules while still prioritizing their health and well-being.

CHAPTER SIX

FLAVORFUL AND HEALING RECIPES FOR BREAKFAST

Energizing Morning Options:

Starting the day with a balanced and energizing breakfast is vital for persons following the Sjogren's Syndrome diet. It sets the tone for the day, delivering the necessary nutrition and energy needed to undertake daily chores.

Here are some delectable and healthful breakfast options intended to satisfy the dietary requirements of those with Sjogren's Syndrome.

A great and nutrient-packed choice is the Berry Bliss Smoothie. Begin by harvesting fresh berries such as blueberries, raspberries, and strawberries.

These berries are not only delicious but also rich in antioxidants, which can help reduce inflammation linked with Sjogren's Syndrome.

44

Combine the berries with a dairy-free milk option like almond or coconut milk for a creamy mouthfeel.

Add a handful of spinach for an added nutritious boost without compromising the flavor. To sweeten, choose a natural sweetener like honey or maple syrup, avoiding processed sugars that may trigger inflammation. Blend the ingredients until smooth, and you have a refreshing and invigorating smoothie ready to launch your day.

Another wonderful choice is the Quinoa Power Bowl. Quinoa is a gluten-free grain that is easy to digest and filled with protein. Begin by cooking the quinoa according to the package instructions. While the quinoa is cooking, sauté a variety of bright veggies such as bell peppers, zucchini, and cherry tomatoes in olive oil. Once the quinoa is finished, combine it with the sautéed vegetables, then top it off with avocado slices for a dose of healthy fats. Season with herbs and spices like turmeric and ginger, known for their anti-inflammatory effects.

This Quinoa Power Bowl not only delivers continuous energy but also enhances general well-being.

For those who want a warm and cozy option, the Ginger Turmeric Oatmeal is a fantastic choice. Oats are an excellent source of fiber, and the combination of ginger and turmeric adds anti-inflammatory properties. Begin by boiling rolled oats in water or a dairy-free milk replacement. Grate fresh ginger and add it to the oats along with a pinch of turmeric. Stir well until the oats are creamy and imbued with the flavors. To increase sweetness, include sliced bananas or a drizzle of pure maple syrup. This steaming bowl of oats is not only relaxing but also nourishing for persons with Sjogren's Syndrome.

Step-by-Step Instructions for Easy Preparation:

Navigating the kitchen can be a daunting endeavor for newbies, but with clear step-by-step directions, creating Sjogren's Syndrome-friendly breakfasts becomes a snap. Let's break down the procedure for the Berry Bliss Smoothie, Quinoa Power Bowl, and Ginger Turmeric Oatmeal.

Berry Bliss Smoothie:

1. Gather Ingredients: Collect fresh berries, dairy-free milk (almond or coconut), spinach, and a natural sweetener (honey or maple syrup).

2. Measure Ingredients: Use one cup of mixed berries, a handful of spinach, and one to two cups of the chosen milk. Add a tablespoon of the sweetener.

3. Blend: Place all ingredients in a blender and blend until smooth. Adjust the thickness by adding more milk if needed.

4. Pour and Enjoy: Pour the smoothie into a glass, and you have a nutritious and pleasant breakfast ready to go.

Quinoa Power Bowl:

1. Prepare Quinoa: Cook quinoa according to package instructions.

2. Sauté Vegetables: While quinoa is cooking, sauté colorful vegetables in olive oil until soft.

3. Combine Ingredients: Mix cooked quinoa with sautéed vegetables, and top with avocado slices.

4. Season: Add turmeric, ginger, and other favorite herbs and spices. Mix well.

5. Serve: Your Quinoa Power Bowl is now ready to be served, giving a delightful and nutrient-packed breakfast.

Ginger Turmeric Oatmeal:

1. Cook Oats: Prepare rolled oats in water or a dairy-free milk replacement.

2. Add Flavors: Grate fresh ginger and add it to the oats along with a pinch of turmeric. Stir thoroughly.

3. Sweeten: Include sliced bananas or a sprinkle of pure maple syrup for sweetness.

4. Mix Well: Ensure the ginger and turmeric are uniformly distributed, infusing the oats with their anti-inflammatory qualities.

5. Enjoy Warm: Your Ginger Turmeric Oatmeal is ready to be eaten, delivering a comforting and healing start to your day.

Chia Seed Parfait:

1. Soak Chia Seeds: Begin by soaking chia seeds in a liquid of your choosing, such as almond milk or coconut milk. Use a ratio of roughly 1/4 cup of chia seeds to 1 cup of liquid. Allow them to sit for at least 30 minutes or overnight until they develop a gel-like consistency.

2. Layer with Fruits: Once the chia seeds have absorbed the liquid, start piling them in a glass or bowl with fresh fruits such as sliced kiwi, mango, or pineapple. These fruits not only give natural sweetness but also contribute vitamins and minerals.

3. Add Crunchy Toppings: Enhance the texture by putting a handful of chopped nuts or seeds on top. Options like almonds, walnuts, or pumpkin seeds provide a delicious crunch and additional nutrition.

4. Sprinkle with Honey: For a touch of sweetness, sprinkle the parfait with a small quantity of honey or agave syrup. This step offers a delicious flavor without compromising the health-conscious parts of the Sjogren's Syndrome diet.

5. Refrigerate and Serve: Let the chia seed parfait refrigerate for at least an hour before serving. This not only chills the parfait but also allows the flavors to mingle. Serve it as a refreshing and nutrient-dense breakfast choice.

Sweet Potato and Spinach Breakfast Hash:

1. Prepare Sweet Potatoes: Peel and dice sweet potatoes into tiny, even pieces. Boil or steam them until they are soft yet firm. This ensures they fry evenly when making the hash.

2. Sauté Vegetables: In a skillet, sauté sliced onions and bell peppers in olive oil until they are softened. Add in fresh spinach and continue cooking until it wilts.

3. Combine with Sweet Potatoes: Mix the sautéed vegetables with the boiling sweet potatoes. Season with salt, pepper, and a dash of paprika for extra taste.

4. Create Wells for Eggs: Make small wells in the hash mixture and crack eggs into each well. Cover the skillet and let the eggs simmer until the whites are set but the yolks remain runny.

5. Garnish and Serve: Garnish the hash with fresh herbs like parsley or chives. Serve immediately, ensuring that the runny egg yolks lend a creamy texture to the Sweet Potato and Spinach Breakfast Hash.

Coconut Flour Pancakes:

1. Combine Dry Ingredients: In a bowl, mix coconut flour, baking powder, and a touch of salt. Coconut flour is a gluten-free alternative that gives a slight sweetness to the pancakes.

2. Add Wet Ingredients: Whisk together eggs, coconut milk, and a tablespoon of melted coconut oil. Slowly integrate the wet ingredients into the dry mixture, stirring until a smooth batter emerges.

3. Cook Pancakes: Heat a non-stick skillet or griddle over medium heat. Spoon small amounts of batter over the surface, spreading it into a circular shape. Cook until bubbles appear on the surface, then turn and cook the other side until golden brown.

4. Serve with Berries: Top the Coconut Flour Pancakes with fresh berries, such as raspberries or blueberries. Berries not only enhance the flavor but also supply antioxidants, helping to the anti-inflammatory part of the Sjogren's Syndrome diet.

5. Drizzle with Maple Syrup: Finish by drizzling a little amount of pure maple syrup over the pancakes. This natural sweetener gives a touch of sweetness without sacrificing the health-conscious approach. Enjoy these fluffy and coconut-flavored pancakes as a lovely breakfast alternative.

CHAPTER SEVEN

NUTRIENT-RICH LUNCH IDEAS

Portable and Satisfying Meals:

When following the Sjögren's syndrome diet, it's crucial to prioritize nutrient-rich, portable, and fulfilling foods during lunch. This is vital, especially for persons struggling with the symptoms of dry mouth and trouble swallowing linked with Sjögren's syndrome. Creating meals that are not only convenient but also packed with important nutrients can make the lunchtime experience more delightful and supportive of overall well-being.

One easy and portable lunch option is a quinoa salad with a variety of bright vegetables. Quinoa is a gluten-free grain that is rich in protein and fiber, giving continuous energy throughout the day. To make this dish even more convenient, cook a batch of quinoa in advance and store it in individual containers in the fridge. When it's time for lunch, simply combine the quinoa with a mix of diced cucumbers, tomatoes, bell peppers, and your favorite herbs. Drizzle with a little vinaigrette made from olive oil, lemon juice, and a bit of salt for extra flavor.

Another portable alternative is a nutrient-dense wrap filled with lean protein, veggies, and a tasty spread. Opt for a whole-grain or gluten-free wrap to suit dietary requirements. Spread a layer of hummus or avocado on the wrap for extra creaminess and healthy fats. Fill it with sliced turkey or chicken, leafy greens, and crisp veggies like carrots and bell peppers. Roll it up tightly and seal it with a toothpick or wrap it in parchment paper for easy handling. This not only assures a substantial lunch but also allows for easy transportation, making it an ideal alternative for individuals on the go.

Incorporating Variety into Your Midday Routine:

Maintaining a wide and varied lunch routine is vital for those with Sjögren's disease, as it helps ensure a broad range of nutrients to maintain general health. Incorporating variety into your midday meals not only eliminates monotony but also gives a larger range of critical vitamins and minerals necessary for treating the symptoms of Sjögren's syndrome.

Start by experimenting with different protein sources. While lean meats like chicken and turkey are wonderful choices, try including plant-based proteins such as beans, lentils, and tofu. These choices not only diversify your food intake but also contribute to a well-balanced and inflammation-reducing diet, which is excellent for those with autoimmune disorders like Sjögren's syndrome.

To add a flash of color and taste to your lunch, explore a rainbow of vegetables. Include a variety of leafy greens, cruciferous vegetables, and colorful peppers to provide a wide assortment of nutrients. A vegetable stir-fry using a variety of colorful veggies can be a simple and pleasurable method to do this. Experiment with different spices and herbs to increase the taste without relying on excessive salt, which may contribute to dehydration.

In addition to varying protein and vegetables, vary your grain selections to incorporate a spectrum of critical elements. Swap typical white rice for brown rice, quinoa, or other whole grains to enhance fiber content and give a continuous flow of energy. Experimenting with different grains not only provides diversity to your lunch but also helps digestive health, a critical component for persons managing autoimmune disorders.

By continuously mixing varied components and trying new recipes, you not only cater to your nutritional demands but also convert your noon meal into a joyful experience. This variety not only leads to better health outcomes but also assists in building a sustainable and enjoyable eating pattern, ensuring that patients with Sjögren's syndrome may maintain a balanced and satisfying diet.

CHAPTER EIGHT

NOURISHING SNACKS FOR SJOGREN'S WARRIORS

Quick and Healthy Bites:

In the realm of Sjogren's Syndrome, maintaining a nutrient-dense diet is paramount to managing symptoms and enhancing overall well-being. Quick and healthy snacks play a crucial role in providing essential nutrients while keeping energy levels stable. For Sjogren's warriors, incorporating snacks that are both convenient and nutritious can be a game-changer.

One go-to option is a delightful fruit and nut medley. Begin by selecting a variety of fresh fruits, such as berries, apples, and grapes, rich in antioxidants that combat inflammation. Combine these with a mix of unsalted nuts like almonds, walnuts, and pistachios, packed with healthy fats and protein. Preparing this snack is as simple as washing and chopping the fruits, and then tossing them with the nuts for a delightful, nutrient-packed treat.

Another quick bite with a nutritional punch is a Greek yogurt parfait. Opt for plain, unsweetened Greek yogurt as the base, as it is not only rich in probiotics that support gut health but also contains protein to keep you feeling satisfied. Layer it with fresh fruits, a drizzle of honey for natural sweetness, and a sprinkle of granola for added crunch. This snack not only caters to the taste buds but also contributes to digestive well-being, a significant consideration for those with Sjogren's Syndrome.

For those on the move, a vegetable and hummus platter is an excellent option. Prepare a variety of colorful veggies like carrots, cucumbers, and bell peppers, and pair them with hummus for a snack that is both hydrating and fulfilling. The vegetables provide essential vitamins and minerals, while hummus adds a dose of protein and healthy fats. This snack requires minimal preparation—simply wash and cut the vegetables and arrange them alongside a bowl of hummus for a quick, nourishing bite.

Snack Ideas that Promote Sustained Energy:

Sustaining energy levels throughout the day is particularly crucial for individuals managing Sjogren's Syndrome. Fortunately, there are snack ideas tailored to achieve just that – offering a steady release of energy without causing blood sugar spikes.

One such option is a trail mix that combines a variety of nuts, seeds, and dried fruits. Begin by selecting almonds, cashews, pumpkin seeds, and dried cranberries or raisins. These ingredients provide a mix of complex carbohydrates, healthy fats, and proteins. Assembling the trail mix involves combining the selected items in a container, ensuring a well-balanced blend. Portion control is key, and packing small servings in advance ensures a convenient and energy-boosting snack is readily available.

Oatmeal energy bites are another stellar choice. These bites are not only delicious but also provide a sustained release of energy. Begin by combining oats, nut butter, honey, and a dash of cinnamon in a bowl. Mix thoroughly and then form bite-sized balls. The oats offer complex carbohydrates, while the nut butter adds healthy fats and protein, creating a well-rounded snack that supports lasting energy. These can be prepared in batches and stored for quick and easy access during snack times.

A smoothie bowl is a versatile and energizing snack that caters to individual taste preferences. Start with a base of frozen fruits like berries or bananas and blend them with Greek yogurt, a splash of milk or a dairy-free alternative, and a handful of spinach for an added nutrient boost. Top the smoothie bowl with granola, nuts, and seeds for added texture and sustained energy. Experimenting with different fruit combinations allows for a personalized snack experience that aligns with both taste preferences and nutritional needs.

Therefore, quick and healthy bites, along with snacks promoting sustained energy, can be seamlessly integrated into the Sjogren's Syndrome diet. By choosing nutrient-dense options and incorporating a variety of flavors and textures, individuals can not only manage their symptoms effectively but also enjoy a diverse and satisfying snacking experience.

CHAPTER NINE

SATISFYING DINNERS FOR SYMPTOM RELIEF

Evening Meals for Symptom Relief

When it comes to crafting satisfying dinners for symptom relief in the context of a Sjogren's Syndrome diet, it's crucial to strike a balance between comfort and nutrition. Evening meals play a pivotal role in not only satiating hunger but also in promoting overall well-being for individuals managing Sjogren's Syndrome. Let's delve into some key components and strategies for creating meals that offer both relief and enjoyment.

Begin by incorporating a variety of nutrient-dense foods into your evening meals. Opt for lean proteins, such as grilled chicken, fish, or tofu, which provide essential amino acids for muscle maintenance and repair. Include a colorful array of vegetables rich in antioxidants, vitamins, and minerals. Leafy greens, bell peppers, and tomatoes can contribute not only to the visual appeal of your plate but also to the reduction of inflammation and oxidative stress associated with Sjogren's Syndrome.

In addition to vegetables, consider incorporating whole grains into your evening meals. Brown rice, quinoa, or whole wheat pasta can serve as excellent sources of fiber, promoting digestive health and aiding in the regulation of blood sugar levels. Fiber-rich foods can also contribute to a feeling of fullness, preventing overeating and supporting weight management—a crucial aspect of overall health for those with Sjogren's Syndrome.

Experiment with herbs and spices to enhance the flavor of your meals without relying on excessive salt or sugar. Turmeric, ginger, and garlic, for instance, not only add depth to your dishes but also possess anti-inflammatory properties that may be particularly beneficial for individuals managing autoimmune conditions like Sjogren's Syndrome.

As you explore various flavor combinations, keep in mind your taste preferences to ensure that your meals are not only nutritious but also enjoyable.

Consider the timing of your evening meals to optimize symptom relief. Aim for a well-balanced dinner that includes a combination of proteins, carbohydrates, and fats. Distribute your caloric intake evenly throughout the evening, allowing for a steady release of energy and preventing blood sugar spikes. This can contribute to stable energy levels, aiding in the management of fatigue—a common symptom experienced by individuals with Sjogren's Syndrome.

In summary, crafting evening meals for symptom relief involves a thoughtful selection of nutrient-dense foods, mindful seasoning, and strategic meal timing. By focusing on a variety of whole foods, incorporating anti-inflammatory ingredients, and paying attention to personal preferences, you can create dinners that not only support your health but also bring satisfaction to your taste buds.

One-Pot Wonders and Easy Cleanup

For those managing Sjogren's Syndrome, the concept of one-pot wonders and easy cleanup dinners can be a game-changer. These approaches not only simplify the cooking process but also minimize the time and effort spent in the kitchen, providing a practical solution for individuals dealing with fatigue and other symptoms associated with the condition.

Begin by selecting recipes that lend themselves well to one-pot cooking. One-pot wonders often involve combining ingredients in a single pot or pan, allowing flavors to meld and minimizing the number of utensils and dishes used during preparation. This approach not only streamlines the cooking process but also facilitates easy cleanup—an appealing prospect for those with Sjogren's Syndrome who may experience fatigue or joint pain.

One classic example of a one-pot wonder is a hearty soup or stew. These dishes typically involve simmering a combination of proteins, vegetables, and grains in a single pot, allowing for the development of rich flavors and a nourishing meal in one container. Consider experimenting with different broth bases, such as vegetable or bone broth, to add depth and nutrition to your one-pot creations.

Another option for easy cleanup is sheet pan dinners. By arranging proteins and vegetables on a baking sheet and roasting them together, you can achieve a well-balanced and flavorful meal with minimal fuss. This approach not only reduces the number of pots and pans used but also allows for easy customization—mix and match your favorite ingredients and seasonings to suit your taste preferences.

To further simplify the cooking and cleanup process, consider investing in quality kitchen tools. Non-stick pots and pans, slow cookers, and instant pots can be valuable additions to your culinary arsenal. These tools not only make cooking more efficient but also make cleanup a breeze, minimizing the physical strain on individuals with Sjogren's Syndrome.

Therefore, one-pot wonders and easy cleanup dinners offer a practical solution for those managing Sjogren's Syndrome. By selecting recipes that embrace simplicity, utilizing versatile cooking methods, and investing in efficient kitchen tools, you can enjoy delicious and nutritious meals with minimal effort and cleanup—making the dining experience more accessible and enjoyable for individuals dealing with autoimmune conditions.

CHAPTER TEN

DESSERTS THAT DELIGHT WITHOUT COMPROMISING HEALTH

Sweet Treats With A Nutritional Twist

Mindful Indulgence For Those With A Sweet Tooth

Creating desserts that delight without compromising health is a wonderful endeavor, especially for individuals following a specific dietary regimen like the Sjogren's Syndrome diet. Sjogren's Syndrome is an autoimmune disorder that primarily affects the moisture-producing glands of the body, leading to symptoms such as dry eyes and mouth. Managing this condition often involves dietary adjustments to alleviate symptoms and promote overall health and well-being.

When it comes to desserts, the key is to find a balance between satisfying your sweet cravings and nourishing your body with ingredients that support your health goals. Fortunately, there are plenty of nutritious alternatives to traditional dessert ingredients that can be incorporated into your sweet treats without sacrificing flavor or texture.

One essential aspect of creating healthier desserts is to focus on natural, whole-food ingredients. Instead of relying on refined sugars and processed flours, opt for sweeteners and flours that are less processed and retain more nutrients.

For example, you can use alternatives like honey, maple syrup, or coconut sugar to sweeten your desserts, as these options contain beneficial nutrients and antioxidants compared to white sugar.

Additionally, choosing whole-grain flour such as whole wheat, almond flour, or oat flour can add fiber, vitamins, and minerals to your desserts while providing a satisfying texture. Experimenting with different flour combinations can also yield unique flavors and textures in your baked goods.

Another strategy for creating healthier desserts is to incorporate fruits and vegetables whenever possible. Fruits like berries, bananas, and apples can add natural sweetness and moisture to your desserts while providing essential vitamins and minerals. You can use fresh, frozen, or even dried fruits depending on your preferences and seasonal availability.

Incorporating vegetables like carrots, zucchini, or sweet potatoes into desserts can also add moisture and nutritional value without compromising taste. For example, grated carrots or zucchini can be added to muffins or cakes to enhance texture and provide a subtle sweetness.

Moreover, pureed sweet potatoes can add richness and creaminess to desserts like pies or puddings while increasing their nutrient content.

When it comes to fats in desserts, choosing healthier options like nuts, seeds, and plant-based oils can enhance both flavor and nutritional value. Instead of using butter or margarine, consider using alternatives like avocado oil, coconut oil, or nut butter to add richness and moisture to your desserts. These options provide beneficial fats that support heart health and can contribute to a satisfying mouthfeel in your sweet treats.

Furthermore, incorporating nuts and seeds into your desserts can add crunch, texture, and a dose of essential nutrients like protein, fiber, and healthy fats.

You can use chopped nuts or seeds as toppings for desserts like yogurt parfaits or oatmeal bowls, or incorporate them into baked goods like cookies or energy bars for added nutrition and flavor.

In addition to choosing nutritious ingredients, it's essential to be mindful of portion sizes when enjoying desserts, especially if you're managing a health condition like Sjogren's Syndrome.

While healthier dessert options can offer nutritional benefits, they still contain calories and should be enjoyed in moderation as part of a balanced diet.

Practical Steps:

1.   **Choose Nutritious Ingredients:** Start by selecting natural, whole-food ingredients like whole-grain flour, natural sweeteners, fruits, vegetables, nuts, and seeds for your desserts.

2.   **Experiment with Flavors:** Explore different flavor combinations by combining fruits, spices, and extracts to create unique and delicious desserts that suit your taste preferences.

3.   **Modify Recipes:** Adapt your favorite dessert recipes to incorporate healthier ingredients and reduce the amount of refined sugars and fats.

4.   **Practice Portion Control:** Be mindful of portion sizes and enjoy desserts in moderation to maintain a balanced diet and manage your health effectively.

5.   **Get Creative:** Don't be afraid to get creative and experiment with new ingredients and techniques to create desserts that delight your taste buds and support your health goals.

By following these practical steps and incorporating nutritious ingredients into your desserts, you can enjoy sweet treats that delight your taste buds without compromising your health, even while adhering to the Sjogren's Syndrome diet.

CHAPTER ELEVEN

CRAFTING A WEEKLY MEAL PLAN

Simplifying the Planning Process:

Embarking on a weekly meal plan tailored to the needs of individuals with Sjögren's syndrome can be a daunting task at first glance, but with a systematic approach, it can be simplified for even the most novice of cooks. The key is to break down the process into manageable steps, making it more approachable and less overwhelming.

Start by creating a basic template for the week. Allocate specific days for meals and snacks, taking into consideration nutritional requirements and preferences. This initial step serves as the foundation for the entire meal plan, providing structure and a clear roadmap. Consider incorporating a variety of foods to ensure a well-balanced diet, keeping in mind the specific dietary recommendations for Sjögren's syndrome.

Next, compile a list of suitable recipes from the "Sjögren's Syndrome Diet Cookbook." Focus on recipes that align with the dietary guidelines for managing Sjögren's syndrome symptoms. Categorize these recipes into breakfast, lunch, dinner, and snacks. This step streamlines the selection process and helps in maintaining a diverse and enjoyable meal plan.

Once the recipes are chosen, make a comprehensive shopping list. Ensure that all the necessary ingredients are included, and cross-check them with the items already available in your kitchen. This organized approach to shopping minimizes the chances of forgetting key ingredients and saves time during meal preparation.

Consider any time constraints and plan meals accordingly. Identify recipes that can be prepared quickly on busy days and reserve more elaborate dishes for when you have extra time. This foresight ensures that the meal plan is practical and sustainable, even with a hectic schedule.

As a final step in simplifying the planning process, be flexible. Life can be unpredictable, and sticking rigidly to a plan may not always be feasible. Allow room for adjustments and substitutions, ensuring that the meal plan remains adaptable to unforeseen circumstances.

Batch Cooking and Preparing for the Week Ahead:

Batch cooking is a game-changer when it comes to implementing a weekly meal plan, especially for those managing Sjögren's syndrome. This efficient approach not only saves time but also ensures that nutritious meals are readily available, reducing the temptation to opt for less healthy alternatives.

Start by selecting recipes that lend themselves well to batch cooking. Look for dishes that can be easily portioned and reheated without compromising taste or texture. Soups, stews, and casseroles are excellent choices as they often improve in flavor after sitting for a day or two.

Once the recipes are chosen, dedicate a specific day to batch cooking. This might be a weekend day or a time when you have a few uninterrupted hours in the kitchen. Make sure to have all the necessary ingredients prepped and ready to go to streamline the process.

Invest in quality storage containers to keep batch-cooked meals fresh and easily accessible throughout the week. Consider labeling containers with the date of preparation to track freshness and rotation. Opt for containers that are both microwave and freezer-safe for added convenience.

When preparing ingredients for batch cooking, keep in mind the principles of the Sjögren's syndrome diet. Focus on incorporating anti-inflammatory and nutrient-dense foods to support overall health. This includes incorporating a variety of colorful vegetables, lean proteins, and healthy fats.

To further optimize your week, consider preparing components of meals in advance. Chop vegetables, marinate proteins, and portion snacks ahead of time.

This proactive approach minimizes the time spent in the kitchen daily, making it more manageable and enjoyable.

Therefore, simplifying the planning process and embracing batch cooking are pivotal steps in successfully implementing a weekly meal plan tailored for Sjögren's syndrome. By breaking down the tasks into manageable steps, even those unfamiliar with meal planning can navigate the process with ease. Batch cooking, in particular, is a practical strategy that not only saves time but also contributes to the consistent adherence to a nutritious and supportive diet. With thoughtful planning and preparation, managing meals for Sjögren's syndrome becomes an attainable and sustainable practice for optimal well-being.

CHAPTER TWELVE

PRACTICAL PREP TIPS FOR NOVICES

Step-by-Step Guidance for Beginners:

Embarking on a journey towards adopting a Sjogren's syndrome diet can seem overwhelming for novices, but breaking it down into manageable steps makes the process much simpler. The first step is understanding the fundamental principles of the Sjogren's syndrome diet, which primarily focuses on reducing inflammation and promoting overall well-being. Begin by familiarizing yourself with the list of foods that are considered beneficial, such as anti-inflammatory fruits and vegetables, lean proteins, and healthy fats.

The second step involves creating a personalized meal plan tailored to your preferences and dietary needs. Start by incorporating small changes into your daily meals, gradually replacing inflammatory foods with healthier alternatives. This approach helps novices transition smoothly without feeling deprived. Experiment with diverse recipes to discover flavors that resonate with your taste buds while adhering to the dietary guidelines.

To facilitate adherence to the Sjogren's syndrome diet, consider meal prepping. Spend some time each week planning and preparing meals in advance, ensuring that you have nutritious options readily available. This not only saves time but also minimizes the temptation to resort to convenience foods that may not align with the dietary recommendations.

Shopping smart is the third crucial step for beginners. Familiarize yourself with the layout of your local grocery store, emphasizing the sections where you can find Sjogren 's-friendly ingredients. Create a detailed shopping list before heading to the store, focusing on fresh produce, whole grains, and lean proteins. Opt for minimally processed foods to avoid hidden additives that could trigger inflammation.

Furthermore, stay hydrated by incorporating plenty of water into your daily routine. Adequate hydration is essential for individuals with Sjogren's syndrome, as it helps combat dryness associated with the condition. Keep a water bottle with you throughout the day to make it easier to meet your hydration goals.

Lastly, seek support from a healthcare professional or a registered dietitian experienced in managing autoimmune conditions. They can provide personalized guidance based on your specific needs, ensuring that your Sjogren's syndrome diet is both effective and sustainable. Regular check-ins with a healthcare professional can help track progress and make adjustments as needed, fostering a sense of accountability and motivation for beginners.

Overcoming Common Challenges in the Kitchen:

Navigating the kitchen with Sjogren's syndrome can present unique challenges, but with a proactive approach, novices can overcome these obstacles and enjoy a fulfilling cooking experience. One common challenge is dealing with dry mouth and difficulty swallowing, which can make eating and cooking uncomfortable. To address this, focus on incorporating moist and soft foods into your diet, such as soups, stews, and smoothies. Additionally, experiment with different cooking techniques like steaming or slow cooking to enhance moisture in your meals.

Another challenge is managing fatigue, a common symptom of Sjogren's syndrome. To overcome this hurdle, prioritize efficiency in the kitchen. Opt for simple recipes with minimal ingredients and preparation time. Consider batch cooking to have ready-made meals available, reducing the need for constant culinary efforts. Delegate tasks when possible and embrace shortcuts, such as pre-cut vegetables or pre-cooked grains, to streamline the cooking process.

For those experiencing joint pain or stiffness, ergonomic kitchen tools can make a significant difference. Invest in utensils with comfortable grips, utilize kitchen gadgets like jar openers or food processors, and arrange your workspace to minimize unnecessary movement.

These adjustments not only alleviate physical strain but also make cooking a more enjoyable experience.

A frequently encountered challenge is the need to avoid certain ingredients, such as gluten or dairy, due to potential sensitivities. Overcome this by exploring alternative ingredients that align with the Sjogren's syndrome diet. Gluten-free grains, dairy substitutes, and flavorful herbs and spices can add variety and excitement to your meals while adhering to dietary restrictions. Familiarize yourself with these substitutes to diversify your culinary repertoire without compromising on taste.

Lastly, be mindful of portion control to maintain a healthy weight, as excessive weight can exacerbate symptoms of Sjogren's syndrome. Use smaller plates to help regulate portion sizes and focus on nutrient-dense foods to meet your nutritional needs without overeating.

By addressing these common challenges head-on and incorporating practical strategies, beginners can navigate the kitchen with confidence, ensuring a positive and sustainable experience on the Sjogren's syndrome diet.

CHAPTER THIRTEEN

SJOGREN'S-FRIENDLY LIFESTYLE HABITS

Beyond the Kitchen: Holistic Approaches to Well-being

When navigating life with Sjögren's syndrome, it's crucial to recognize that dietary choices are just one aspect of managing symptoms. A holistic approach that encompasses various lifestyle factors is key to achieving overall well-being. Beyond the kitchen, incorporating regular physical activity into your routine is paramount. Engaging in low-impact exercises, such as walking, swimming, or yoga, not only contributes to maintaining a healthy weight but also helps alleviate joint pain commonly associated with Sjögren's.

In addition to physical activity, stress management plays a pivotal role in holistic well-being. Chronic stress can exacerbate Sjögren's symptoms, so adopting stress-reduction techniques is essential. Mindfulness meditation, deep breathing exercises, and progressive muscle relaxation are effective methods to incorporate into your daily routine. These practices not only promote mental calmness but also positively impact your immune system, contributing to better overall health.

Adequate sleep is another often overlooked but critical component. Sjögren's syndrome can cause fatigue, making quality sleep even more vital. Establishing a consistent sleep schedule, creating a relaxing bedtime routine, and optimizing your sleep environment are practical steps to improve sleep quality. This holistic approach, encompassing exercise, stress management, and adequate sleep, empowers individuals with Sjögren's to enhance their overall well-being beyond dietary considerations.

Incorporating Mindful Practices into Daily Life

Mindful practices go beyond diet and exercise; they involve cultivating a heightened awareness of your body and mind. For those navigating Sjögren's syndrome, incorporating mindfulness into daily life can significantly contribute to symptom management and overall quality of life.

To begin with, start your day with a few minutes of mindfulness meditation. Find a quiet space, sit comfortably, and focus on your breath. This simple practice sets a positive tone for the day, promoting a sense of calmness that can carry through challenging moments. As a novice, guided meditation apps or videos can be invaluable resources, providing step-by-step instructions to make the process more accessible.

Mindful eating is another powerful practice to integrate into your routine. Instead of rushing through meals, take time to savor each bite, paying attention to textures and flavors. This not only enhances your dining experience but also promotes better digestion. Additionally, mindful eating helps you tune in to your body's hunger and fullness cues, preventing overeating—a common challenge for individuals with Sjögren's.

Incorporating mindfulness into daily activities, such as walking or washing dishes, can further enhance your overall well-being. By staying present in the moment, you can reduce stress and anxiety, which are often heightened in individuals with Sjögren's syndrome. As you cultivate these mindful practices, you'll find that they seamlessly integrate into your daily life, providing valuable tools for managing the challenges associated with Sjögren's.

CONCLUSION

Empowering You on Your Sjogren's Journey

This comprehensive guide is designed to simplify your culinary experience while addressing the unique needs of those managing Sjogren's Syndrome. Whether you're a seasoned chef or a novice in the kitchen, this cookbook aims to make the process enjoyable, educational, and, most importantly, beneficial to your health.

Empowering individuals on their journey with Sjogren's Syndrome through a dedicated diet cookbook is a commendable initiative. This endeavor is not just a collection of recipes but a comprehensive guide designed to provide practical and achievable steps for individuals grappling with this autoimmune condition. By delving into the contents of the "Sjogren's Syndrome Diet Cookbook," it becomes evident that the primary focus is on imparting knowledge, promoting healthy habits, and making the dietary transition as seamless as possible.

The cookbook strategically begins by elucidating the fundamentals of Sjogren's Syndrome, ensuring that readers, especially novices, gain a thorough understanding of the condition. It breaks down the intricacies of how diet can play a pivotal role in managing symptoms and improving overall well-being. This foundational knowledge serves as a solid platform for individuals who may be new to the concept of dietary intervention for autoimmune disorders.

Moving forward, the cookbook thoughtfully outlines a step-by-step approach to adopting a Sjogren's-friendly diet. It doesn't overwhelm readers with a multitude of information but rather takes a methodical and demonstrative approach. Novices are guided through a journey that begins with basic dietary changes and gradually progresses to more advanced strategies. This staged progression ensures that individuals can adapt to the new dietary habits at their own pace, minimizing confusion and maximizing adherence.

Practicality is a key theme woven throughout the cookbook, and this is particularly evident in the variety of recipes offered. The cookbook doesn't just present a list of foods to avoid and include; it goes the extra mile by providing a diverse array of delicious and nourishing recipes. These recipes are not only tailored to suit the specific needs of individuals with Sjogren's but are also designed with simplicity in mind. Each recipe is accompanied by clear instructions, and the ingredients are readily accessible, making it easy for novices to replicate the dishes without feeling overwhelmed.

Furthermore, the cookbook doesn't just stop at providing recipes; it equips readers with valuable tools for meal planning and preparation. Novices are guided on how to create well-balanced meals that not only cater to their nutritional requirements but also align with the principles of a Sjogren 's-friendly diet. This hands-on approach instills confidence in individuals who may initially feel daunted by the prospect of revamping their dietary habits.

An integral aspect of the cookbook is its emphasis on customization. Recognizing that each individual's journey with Sjogren's Syndrome is unique, the cookbook encourages readers to tailor the dietary guidelines to their specific needs.

In essence, the "Sjogren's Syndrome Diet Cookbook" stands as a beacon of empowerment for individuals navigating the complexities of this autoimmune condition. It provides a well-crafted roadmap that leads novices through a transformative journey toward better health. By demystifying the intricacies of dietary management and offering practical, guided steps, the cookbook not only fosters optimal adherence but also fosters a sense of empowerment and control over one's health. Through this resource, individuals with Sjogren's Syndrome are not just recipients of information but active participants in their well-being, equipped with the knowledge and tools to thrive on their unique journey.

MY GRATITUDES

Dear Valued Readers and Supporters,

I hope this message finds you well. I am writing to express my deepest gratitude to both God and each one of you for the overwhelming support and positive response to my book. Your encouragement and enthusiasm have truly touched my heart, and I am immensely thankful for the journey we are on together.

I believe that every success is a result of collaboration and support from various sources. First and foremost, I want to acknowledge the divine guidance and inspiration that led me to create this cookbook. Without the grace of God, this endeavor would not have been possible.

To my cherished readers, your commitment to exploring healthier dietary options for managing your crises has been both inspiring and humbling. Your trust in this book" means the world to me, and I am honored to be part of your journey toward improved health and well-being.

Also, I am reaching out to kindly request your valuable feedback on this book. Your thoughts and insights are crucial in helping me enhance and serve you better, ensuring that it continues to meet your needs effectively. Please take a moment to share your thoughts by rating and writing reviews on platforms where the book is available.

Your reviews not only provide me with invaluable feedback but also play a significant role in assisting others in making informed choices. By sharing your experiences, you contribute to a community that values health and wellness, creating a positive impact on countless lives.

Additionally, I encourage you to share this book with your friends, family and loved ones.

Together, we can extend the reach of this promising resource, offering support and guidance to those who may benefit from it. Having this knowledge and seeking medical advice from your specialist I anticipate a turnaround for us.

Once again, thank you from the depths of my heart for your unwavering support. I am committed to continually improving and serving you better. Let us continue this journey together, promoting health, well-being, and a shared sense of community.

With sincere appreciation,

 [Emmy Brooks]

Author, "SJOGREN'S SYNDROME DIET COOKBOOK"

www.ingramcontent.com/pod-product-compliance
Lightning Source LLC
Chambersburg PA
CBHW070749290526
45795CB00002B/537